Ancient Tonics and Diets

Traditional Food Items and Recipes Which Will Keep You Strong, Healthy, and Vigorous

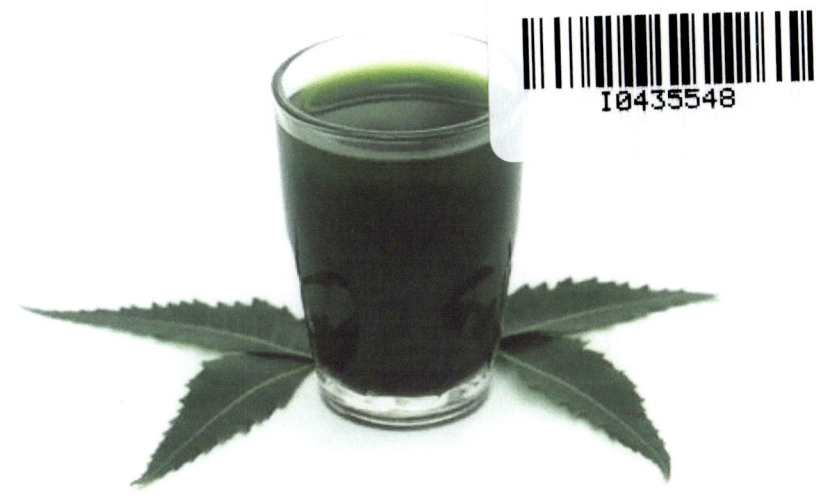

Health Learning Series

Dueep Jyot Singh

Mendon Cottage Books

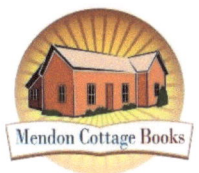

JD-Biz Publishing

Our books are available at

1. Amazon.com
2. Barnes and Noble
3. Itunes
4. Kobo
5. Smashwords
6. Google Play Books

Download Free Books!

http://MendonCottageBooks.com

Table of Contents

Introduction

When I was doing a bit of research on ancient Eastern philosophies, and lifestyles, as well as on diets, which kept them happy and healthy, I noticed that there were a number of recipes which have been disregarded by mankind, or possibly have been forgotten because either they were written in hieroglyphics or in Sanskrit or in some ancient language.

So this book is going to tell you all about the remedies I collected from my own library, and from these ancient books, on tonics as well as food items, and how you are going to eat them in order to keep healthy and happy for as long as you live.

Many of these food items were eaten by human beings and then with the passing of time, they began to be forgotten as a normal dietary intake. So let us start with food items for growing children, adolescents, and people doing physical labor.

Energy giving foods for youngsters and those doing physical work

When I was reading General Lew Wallace's Book, <u>Ben Hur</u>, I was interested in the energy giving horse food, Sheik Alderim ordered to be given to his desert treasures. Nowhere did I see black gram. I was astonished. General Wallace, being an American war hero, should have known that this was one of the most important energy giving foods being given to horses since ancient times.

Instead, they were given cut grass, wheat, and oats. Apart from that, they were given 14 pounds of hay and about 12 pounds of barley, corn, and oats.

This was the prescribed diet for one horse during one day. This naturally meant that they were spending a lot of time and energy lugging food and water to horses, and most of the times, these horses starved because they could not get adequate food and water supply.

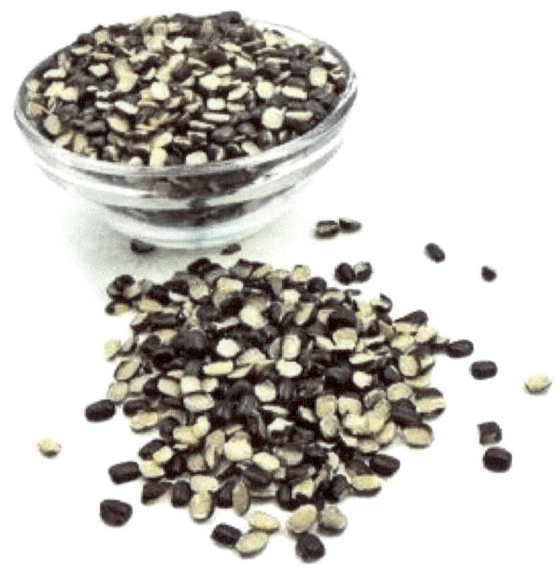

Possibly these generals did not know about ancient food items being given to horses in the shape of black gram. If they are good enough to give horses enough of energy to conquer the ancient world in Alexander's and Caesar's time, they are good enough to give you that much of energy throughout the day. It is also known as the garbanzo bean. We are talking about the black bean here, and not the white one used in the making of hummus, even though it is equally proteinaceous.

https://en.wikipedia.org/wiki/Chickpea

For this, we are going to take 25 g of black beans, clean them thoroughly, and wash them. Put them in 125 g of water and soak them overnight. The next morning, you are going to eat them raw, for breakfast by chewing them properly. Having been soaked overnight, you can munch on them. This is an acquired taste, because they are going to have a taste of well, beans soaked overnight!

Drink the water, because it is going to have all the minerals in it, obtained during the soaking. This is going to clear your system and all the minerals are going to be absorbed in your system. I was looking around in the stores, and found that these garbanzo beans normally come in a creamish color or in a reddish brown color. Pure black chickpeas were rather difficult to find, but even if they are in a reddish-brown color, do not worry, the energy quotient is exactly the same of what you would get, when you were feeding this to your pet horse.

If you really want lots of energy, you can add a little bit of honey to that water, and then you are set for the day. You can go and work hard outside, without worrying about getting tired or thinking of a diminished energy quotient. Leave some for grazing at night.

In a couple of days, you are going to increase the quantity of the chickpeas from 25 g to 50 g depending on how much energy you need. In fact, in ancient times, it was said that if a person was flagging in his virility – this seems to be a perpetual age-old fear, he was immediately fed this by his wife, followed with a glassful of milk and fresh homemade butter on bread. It supposedly increased the potency of a man, and reassured him that he would be the provider of sons!

In the same way, you could eat these at night too, after you have had your dinner, drink it down with the water, and you are going to have absolutely no problem with constipation or any other problem ever.

However, there are some restrictions for those people who are not allowed to eat black gram. If you have a delicate digestive system, do not eat them. Do not eat them if you suffer from chronic flatulence.

Incidentally, I get over this problem, because I cannot do without spicy chickpeas, by adding lots of ginger to the dish while cooking. This counteracts the flatulence problem. Also I make sure that I have lots of sliced up unpeeled oranges on the table, when I am eating spicy food, so that I can allow the orange peels to help with indigestion and prevent flatulence!

Black Gram Sprouts

Any chickpea or bean is going to be excellent sprouting material and more nutritious when the leaves are 2 – 3 in number.

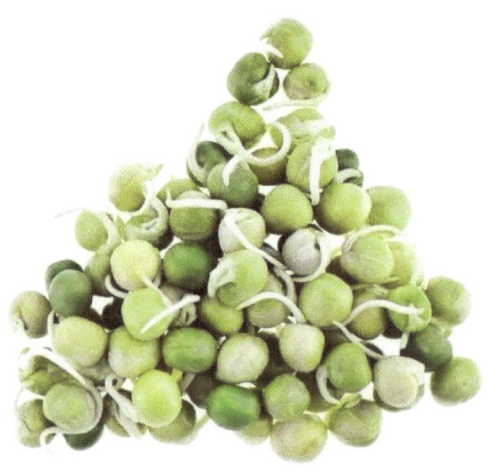

Just like mung sprouts, black gram sprouts can be sprouted really easily. They are rich in minerals and not only help in the growth of your muscles and tissues, but also they are excellent preventatives of diseases.

If you are taking them regularly as a breakfast, you are going to find an increase in muscular mass, especially if you support it with physical labor. This also has a lot of vitamin C so that means you are not going to suffer from coughs and colds.

Also, since ancient times, people knew that a regular intake of these particular grams would keep your lungs healthy, so you would never suffer from tuberculosis. It also reduced the amount of cholesterol from your blood and kept your circulatory system going strong. Also, if you have a tendency to suffer from any heart ailments, try adding this black gram in large quantities to your daily diet. You are going to be surprised at the visible benefits accrued from this healthy natural food intake.

So how do you sprout these black gram? Wash and clean them and soak them in just enough water which can be absorbed by the seeds, early in the morning. By night time, the water will have been absorbed. You are now going to transfer the seeds to a thick natural fabric, like cotton cloth, which has been well moistened. You can also tie them up in a cloth bag and hang them up somewhere in the kitchen.

It takes 12 hours for them to sprout in the summer and anywhere between 18 to 24 hours for them to sprout in the winter. Remember to keep them moisturized, but not soaking in water. You are going to see the little sprouts putting out leaves within 48 hours. Consider this to be the best and healthiest breakfast food ever thought of by man.

Nowadays, they are adulterated with salt-and-pepper to taste, rock salt, ginger, lemon juice, garlic salt, and red pepper, and if you want to try it this way, I would suggest eating unadulterated sprouts for breakfast and seasoned with spices sprouts throughout the day, whenever you want an energy boost.

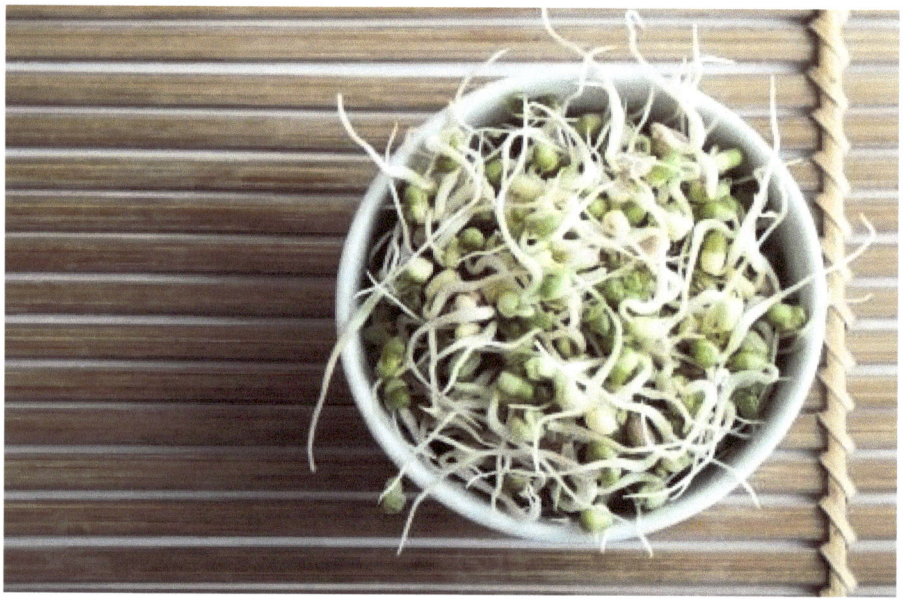

They are also delicious, healthy, nutritious and energy giving. In fact, any seed, which is edible and which has been sprouted is going to be an instant energy booster, because of the green leaves and germinating sprout.

Figs

This was, of course, one of the most important food items in the ancient world, especially in the Mediterranean region, Egypt, Africa and in the Middle East.

I was looking through ancient Roman recipes, just to see what Lucullus – as in *a feast fit for Lucullus , lucullan being a synonym for gastronomic delights, lavish, and extravagant* – on his family estate in Tuscany ate and he seemed to be munching on figs, as often as possible.

Well, the ancients knew that all you had to do when you thought you were growing old, was to eat 2 – 3 dried figs for breakfast on top of which, you would drink it down with a glass full of milk in which you had added 2 – 3 tablespoonfuls of honey.

Bye-bye, old age. Hello energy, vigor, and strength.

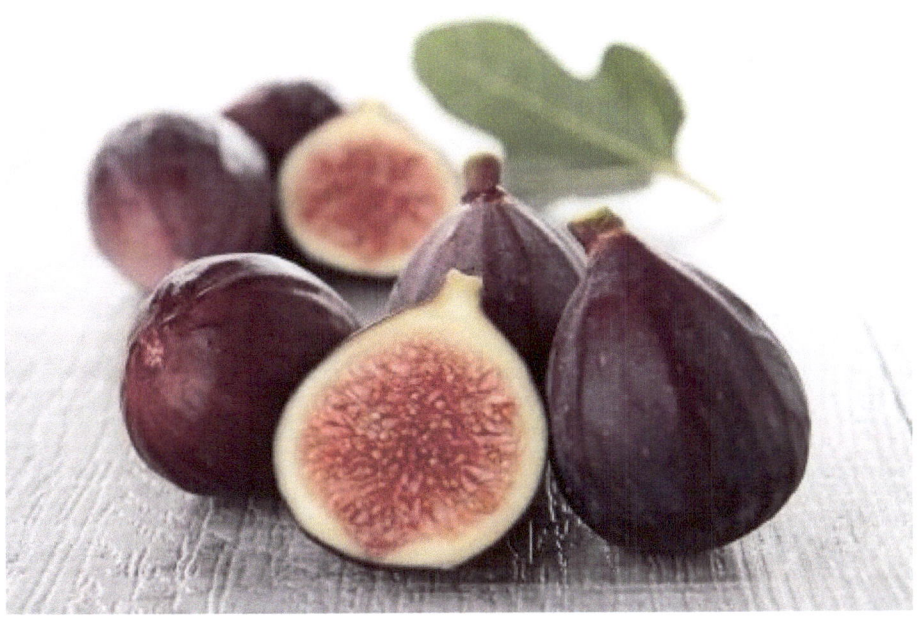

Ancient wise men knew that figs were excellent for the stomach, to cure stomach ailments, constipation, and ailments in the blood. So anybody who was lethargic, or suffered from anemia or problems in the stomach brought about through overeating and did not have energy to do any sort of work were immediately hauled up to the wise man of the town who would feed them with milk and figs.

Also, the women of ancient times were considered to be very beautiful, fair of face, because they ate figs regularly. Also, people suffering from respiratory problems, especially asthma and TB – tuberculosis was an ancient disease – was put on a diet of figs and grapes with milk, butter, buttermilk, and honey to restore him to good health.

With the passing of time, people would find their teeth falling out, and they could not munch on the figs. So these figs were put overnight in water, in just enough water that could be absorbed properly into the figs, which would feed the toothless elders at breakfast. And then they would be given the soft pulpy flesh of figs in the morning, with milk to keep them healthy and chirpy.

In the same way, anybody suffering from hemorrhoids was fed figs, 2 – 3 figs were placed in water in the morning, and fed to them at night. Then 2 – 3 of the figs were soaked overnight, and fed to them in the morning. This took about one month to cure the hemorrhoids, but this ensured a permanent cure.

Health Giving Food for the Elderly

Why are so many of our elders suffering from health related diseases, especially senility? This was definitely not the problem in ancient times, if you go by historical books, when the elders kept up their steady physical, mental, emotional, and spiritual guidance of the youngsters of the town even when they were old and gray.

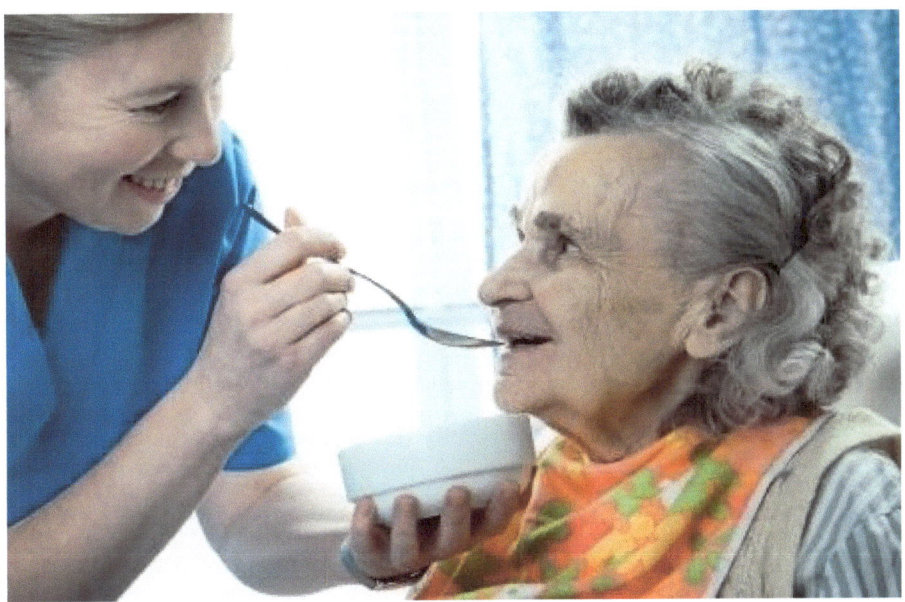

One of the reasons why they kept healthy was because of the attitude towards the elders at that time. These elders were considered to be important and revered parts of society. They were not considered to be human beings who had to be hidden away from public view, just because they were old.

This unfortunately with the passing of time has become a deplorable part of society, when the elderly are considered to be burdens on their family and heavy responsibilities.

The food, which was given to these elders along with the fig and milk diet which I told you above, also included 2 walnuts, 4 almonds, – these soaked overnight, – and 7 raisins. You added them to your breakfast while you still had your teeth, and when you hit your fifties and sixties, so that your brain had enough brainpower to keep working when you hit your seventies and eighties.

When you began losing your teeth, you could grind up these together and feed them to your elders or take them yourself with a glass full of milk in which you had added 4 teaspoons full of honey.

They would then never suffer from physical or mental debilitation of any kind. The only thing is that you would have to take care of them well into their nineties and more, because the ancients went way beyond Man's allocated age of 3 score and 10 because of his sensible diet. This figs diet, along with the dry fruit were particularly efficient in the wintertime, when they needed plenty of warmth, especially due to lowered physical resistance and susceptibility to diseases.

If the elders suffered from constipation, they were given 2 – 3 figs to eat, along with the milk and dry fruit, but not if they suffered from diabetes.

Traditional Health Giving Foods for Children

Date- honey "Chew"

I have long been fascinated by the diet of the Middle East, especially the desert area, where for centuries people survived on fare, which we now considered to be emergency and energy giving rations for the Army!

Dates were an important part of this diet. So I asked some of my Lebanese friends whether they could give me some traditional old recipes for energy which were passed down the ages and which included dates. They did not know any. "Ask your grandma," I growled.

When they stopped laughing because I expected their grandmas to be still living, I told them that mine was – she was at that time – and they blinked. She was 94 and still going strong. So that meant our traditional ancient diet was capable of giving our elders plenty of longevity and energy enough to bully their great-grandchildren in the most autocratic timeworn tradition of grandmas all over the world.

So that put them on their mettle. And here is a traditional recipe coming down straight from the Persian Gulf with dates and coconuts in it.

For this, you are going to get together one part of seedless dates, 2 parts dried grated coconut, and 3 parts rock candy/honey is better. Grate all of them together and make them into a powder. Put this in a glass bottle.

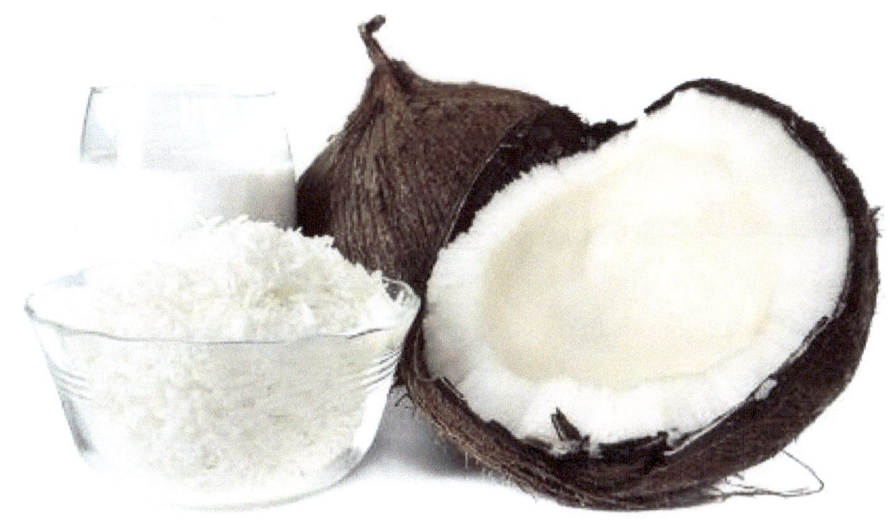

This is an excellent breakfast for your youngsters. Just give them 2 tablespoons full for breakfast everyday. And if they want anything sweet during the day, they can have half a tablespoonful, just as a reward for being particularly good.

Remember not to feed them any liquid for a little while after they have taken this energy boosting tonic. That would not be very difficult in the Middle East, where thousands of years ago, there was a scarcity of water in desert areas and children had learned to do without it. But they drank plenty of milk. Your children are also going to drink milk, but not immediately after their 2 teaspoonfuls of coconut and dates. Give your system at least 2 hours to digest and assimilate the coconut, dates, and honey.

Try this in the winter, especially if your child is prone to winter-based diseases, tonsillitis, coughs, colds, and so on. You can also eat it yourself to get a stronger immune system, thanks to the honey and the dates.

Apples and Carrots for Ladies

Best Food to Reduce and Increase Weight

For millenniums ladies have been very worried about the feminine concept of beauty. In ancient times, a well-rounded figure was considered to be really beautiful. Today, all of them are stick insects because they are not going to eat in a healthy manner because horrors, they may become really fat. Sadly enough, this trend is the reason why so many youngsters are totally unhealthy and that is going to have a detrimental effect on the health of the future generations to come.

Well, this is where I am going to use just these 2 items apples and carrots, especially in the winter, both to reduce weight and to increase weight.

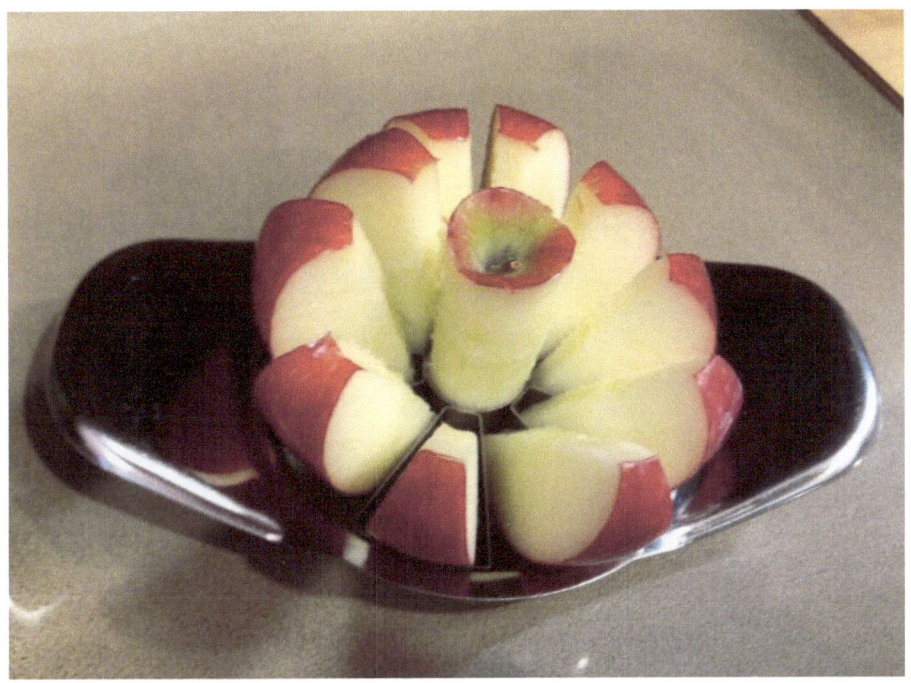

If you want to reduce weight – remember that apples and carrots should never be peeled when you are eating them. Most of the energy giving minerals are under the peels of a large number of vegetables out there and be throw away these nutritious peels because we are more interested in the aesthetic looks of the finally prepared dish that which should not be spoiled with potato peels peeping through the gravy.

Anyway, do not peel your apples and carrots. Grate them separately. Now eat them as many as you can for your breakfast on an empty stomach. You need at least 200 g combined of these 2 items. Let us say 2 1/2 apples and 3 carrots.

Do not eat anything else for about 2 hours after this meal. Try this out and find yourself with a clear complexion, healthy system, and total energy boost.

In the same manner, if you want to increase your weight, you are going to take this 200 g weight of grated apples and carrots, after your lunch. You are going to be eating your lunch with those items which you have been advised by your dietitian for a weight increase after he has checked up that you are not suffering from any possible health causes for a weight loss.

Traditional Food for Babies

My grandfather often recounted to us youngsters that the moment I was born, he in keeping with long time honored Eastern tradition had told the nurses in the military hospital not to give me the first "lick" of honey. The honors were to be left to him as the proud grandpa of his firstborn grandchild.

That was because traditionally it was said that the child's nature "went" on the person who gave the child the first meal before it was given its first feeding of mother's milk.

He wanted a rough and tough little kid. He did not want me to grow up hustling and bustling and hundred percent disciplined and 110% efficient like those spick and span military nurses! They giggled in answer. They understood the value of the first "lick", and took this request to be a part and parcel of their daily routine.

Also, it was said that that little bit of honey given to the baby would get it through the trauma of being born into a thoroughly alien world!

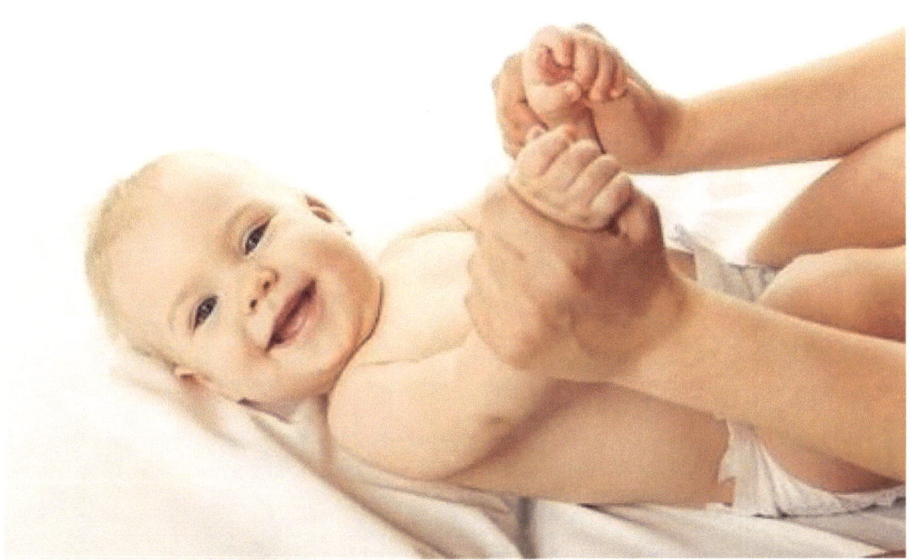

This is a ancient belief in the East. And that is why he was there to feed me a little bit of honey with a clean finger, the moment I entered the world, and had been cleaned up, weighed, and measured and wrapped up in clean cloth. With that, he also breathed a prayer of protection on this new being and blessings.

Traditionally, this prayer requested the Gods to bless the new born soul and any evil upon it being taken upon the head of the blessing giver – in this case, my grandfather.

Incidentally, I found out that this tradition was followed in many parts of the world since ancient times. That was because life was so precarious and survival was difficult, that a child needed all the help that it could get. And that included honey and blessings and help from the Gods.

So be a child heathen, pagan 10,000 years ago or a child born in a modern civilization in the twentieth century, the innate instinct for protection would remain the same in the elders. It will never be removed in human beings.

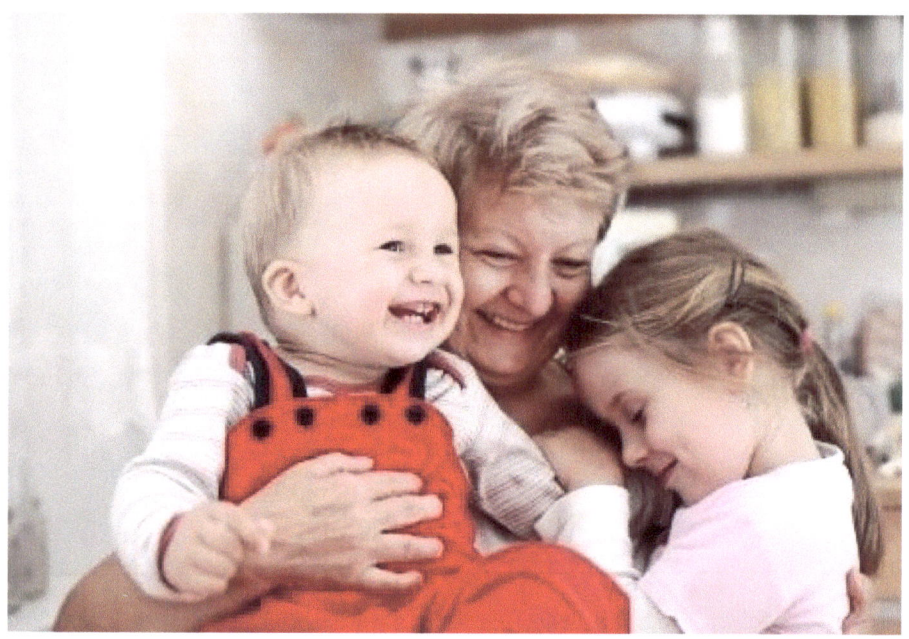

A Grandma with her happy and healthy little babies

In ancient times, it would be the duty of the elders of the tribe to look towards the health and well-being of the little ones while the young children and adults did the rest of the daily work.

Mothers Milk and Colostrum

This little child would of course be fed mother's milk. That would of course include the first mother's milk known as colostrum. I saw in some news reports somewhere, that nurses, by know it all doctors, were told to tell mothers to remove the colostrum beforehand, and not feed it to the babies. Thus depriving the baby with the most powerful and natural source of proteins, antibodies, and immunoglobins, as well as minerals, ever produced by nature.

But then there is some pompous doctor somewhere with an inflated sense of self-importance with nothing to recommend him, but a string of letters behind his name, who definitely knows more than everybody else in the world, because he said so. And people listen to him.

But then he is just building up his practice because those little sickly babies are going to come to him for treatment because they were being deprived of essential, important, and necessary antibodies at birth.

I was also shocked to see colostrum being sold in the form of tablets. This is supposed to be the latest thing and women have begun accepting this idea without using their own common sense, having being encouraged by the doctors to do so? *That means you are feeding your child antibodies and immunoglobulins taken from some other mother, instead of that which he would get naturally from his own mother.*

Think about that.

What absolutely potentially harmful and dangerous thing will the pharmaceutical companies think of next? But they are there to make money at the expense of your health.

So wake up, especially if you are a new mother. Who took away the colostrum and under which excuse? Who told you not to feed your baby colostrum, when you brought your little one home? Who told you that breast-feeding was not a good option, especially if you were worried about your beauty and figure and you had better feed your baby expensive bottled food with energy supplements. And he would recommend those brands to you.

Golly, gadzooks, I am speechless. You have come a long way, baby, being harmed by your own ignorant mother with lots of help from your doctor. God Help You.

So remember, mothers milk, + colostrum + when he was around 4 months old, the grandmother of the tribe would begin feeding him one almond soaked overnight and in the morning made into a very thin paste on a stone with a little bit of milk.

The paste should be as smooth as silk without any lumps because the baby does not have teeth to chew upon pieces of almond. To this would be added just a little bit of honey. Then grandma would put her clean finger into the paste and feed the little baby this, first thing in the morning on an empty stomach, gently, and slowly.

You would want to make sure that the almond is a sweet one so taste a little bit before you soak it overnight. Never feed anyone a bitter almond unless, of course, you want to get rid of them permanently. Bitter almond has potentially lethal prussic acid in it.

The honey was there to give him plenty of immunity. The almond was there to encourage his physical and mental growth by leaps and bounds.

Energy Giving Foods to Helping Increase Muscle Mass

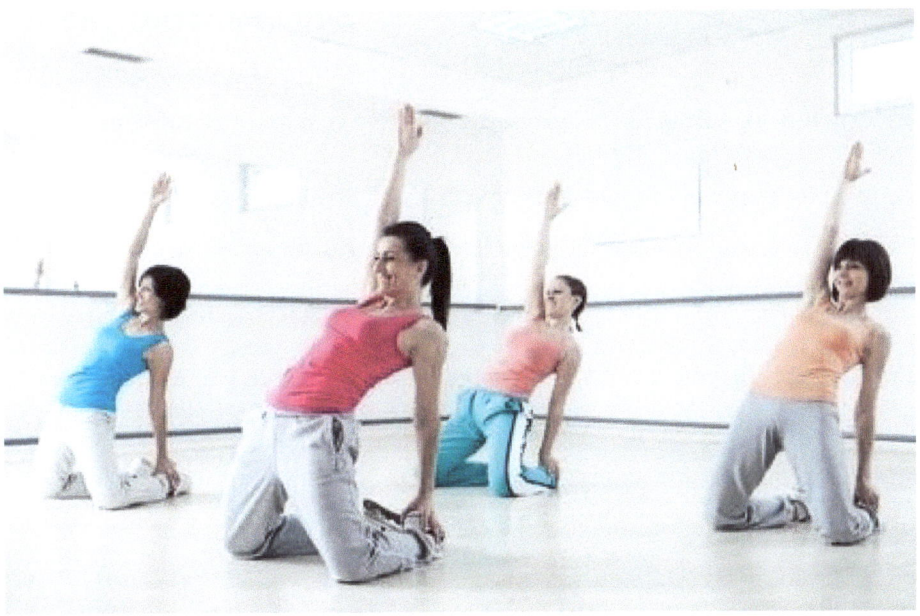

Physical exercise of any kind should also be supported with a good natural diet to get more positive muscle mass.

Date Pudding

This healthy food recipe was told to me by an old lady, who made sure that this breakfast was fed to her children every day. These children were strong, healthy and had an extremely enviable amount of energy. But then she fed them two dates boiled in 2 1/2 glasses of milk.

When the milk was reduced to half its quantity, she would take it off the heat and then she would put 2 spoons full of either date sugar/brown sugar cane sugar – this is the traditional molasses/or honey if she had any. Drink it, when the boiled milk is at room temperature.

If you did not want to boil the milk, you could put dates in the milk and drink it down with honey. This is the best diet to give you muscle mass and energy. It is excellent for people suffering from respiratory problems.

No wonder they could manage to live in the desert area with all those winds blowing and not bother about particles of sand causing problem in the respiratory system.

But here are the precautions which you are going to take when you drink this date milk. This is done only in the winter because it causes plenty of warmth in the body. You are going to do this treatment for just 2 or 3 weeks. If you drink this at nighttime, make sure that you do not drink any water, after that for the next 2 hours.

Here is one beneficial side effect of this drink. If you find yourself with a croaky and harsh voice, this is going to soothe in your throat and make your voice soft, smooth, and gentle. Never eat more than 4 dates at one time, your system cannot take it.

Date Milk

The date milk remedy I told you above is going to be made in this manner. You are going to soak 2 dates overnight in just enough water which is going to be soaked up in the dates. The next morning, remove the seed and throw it away. Now boil them in a glass full of milk. When you have seen that it has been boiled a little, to your satisfaction allow to cool and drink it up.

With this diet you are going to find yourself as hungry as a desert lion. This is also excellent for your digestive system. If you have a baby who wets the bed, just boil a date in 250 g of milk and feed it to the baby when it is cool. This is excellent for elders also who are suffering from incontinency with the passing of time. Do this once a day for 4 days, and you are going to see visible improvements and a permanent and final cure. For elders, you may need to do this treatment for a couple of more days until their system begins to grow stronger again.

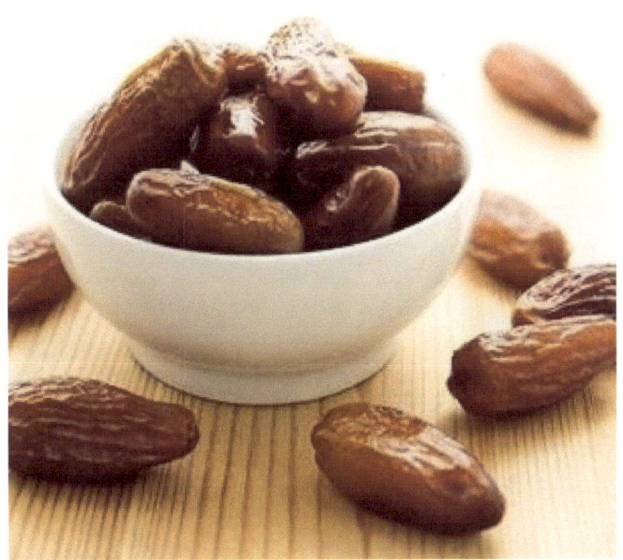

For people suffering from tuberculosis, and other chronic diseases, they were fed the date milk pudding for 40 days, early in the morning and just before they went to sleep until they were cured completely. This is of course an ancient time-tested and timeworn remedy.

Natural Blood Providers

There are plenty of foodstuffs out there, which provide you with red blood corpuscles. So here are some of them.

The best red blood corpuscles providers in the world are grapes. No wonder all the ancients drank such large quantities of grape wine. No one heard of them suffering from anemia, ever.

Black Raisins/sultanas – you are going to take 10 – 12 black

sultanas and soak them overnight. After 12 hours, chew them up first thing in the morning. Do this for 2 – 4 weeks and see the difference. This is also excellent for those people suffering from nosebleed.

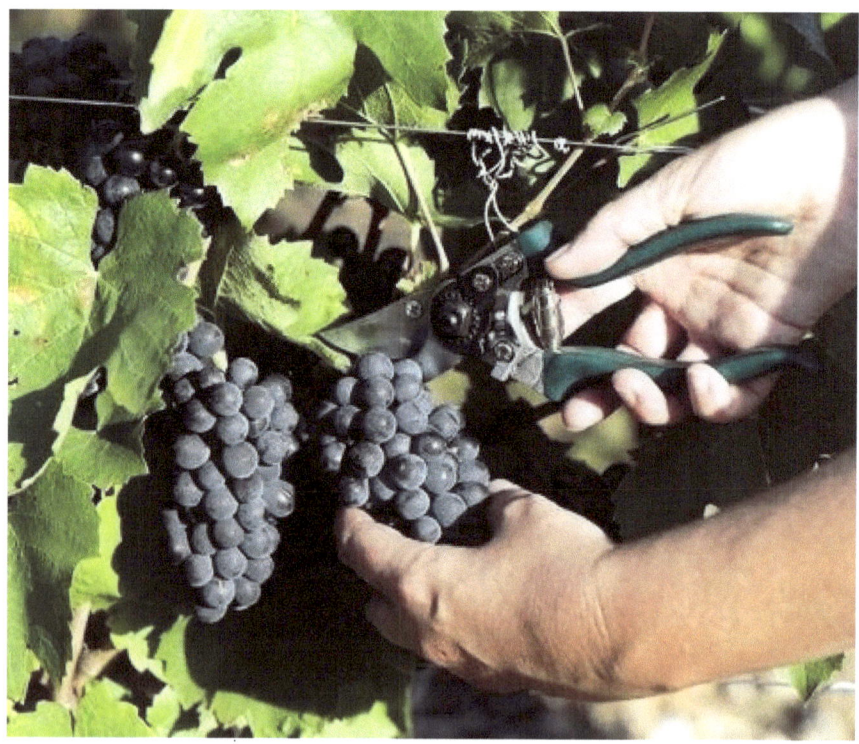

Ordinary raisins – you are going to take 24 – 30 of these raisins, wash them in warm water early in the morning and then drink them in a glass full of milk. Allow them to soak for an hour. Drink up this milk along with the raisins.

Cold Feet and Hands/Bad Circulation

This is excellent for those people who suffer from cold feet and hands; especially in the winter and even if your circulation is sluggish. This is when you are going to try the dry raisin treatment with any of the reasons given above.

Grape juice –

Take 25 g of grape juice and drink it half an hour before lunch and dinner. Try this treatment for 2 weeks. This is going to rejuvenate you, it is considered to be the best tonic for toning up your system, preventing headaches, and digestion related problems, and even heart related problems.

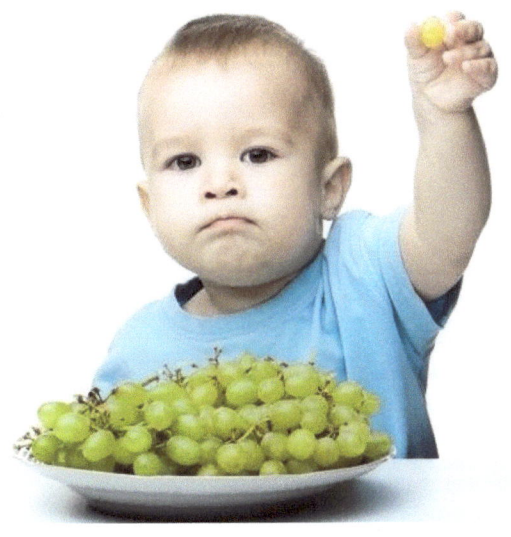

This grape juice is going to be made from fresh grapes. It is also going to increase the body mass. If you have a baby in the family, give him grapes to eat if he can chew foods. If he is just a little baby, give him two spoonfuls of grape juice, with his evening dinner or in the evening. Also, it is going to heal your baby's system. So if he has any obstruction in his little stomach preventing proper elimination, the grape juice is going to clear it.

Women should increase the grape intake in their diets, just as a matter of course, to keep healthy and energetic throughout their lives.

Nearly all the vitamins are present in grapes, especially those belonging to vitamin B complex. Remember that vitamin B complex can never be obtained through supplements, however much your doctor tells you otherwise or the pharmaceutical companies do. These like other important minerals, vitamins, and proteins are obtained from natural foods.

So what would you like to eat, natural foods, giving you natural vitamins or those expensive supplements manufactured in a lab somewhere by a multimillion dollar pharmaceutical company?

Also, if you do not have enough red blood corpuscles in your body, you are going to find yourself suffering from joint ache, swelling in your joints, high and low blood pressure and even tension.

More grapes in your diet means no more stomach cramps.

Remember not to take grapes, raisins, and other dried grape products, if you suffer from diabetes.

Here are some other ancient healthy techniques, which are going to help you keep healthy. These include chewing your food so much, as if you are a bovine until you "drink" it down with absolutely no solid particle of food in your mouth and the mouthful is well mixed with saliva.

Along this, here is one tip given to me about 2 decades ago, when I wanted to give a unit of blood in a blood donation drive, organized by the Lions Club in our city, for community service. They took a sample of my blood from my finger and checked for the RBC count.

I was shocked to hear that I was badly anemic. I was immediately told to drink 125 g of spinach juice by grinding up raw spinach and putting 125 g of water in it for the next 2 weeks and then come again in the next drive to take place after 3 months.

I came home and told my grandmother in a woebegone voice that "they said that I did not have enough of good blood in me." She having served in the Second World War as a Lieutenant- nurse knew everything about anemia.

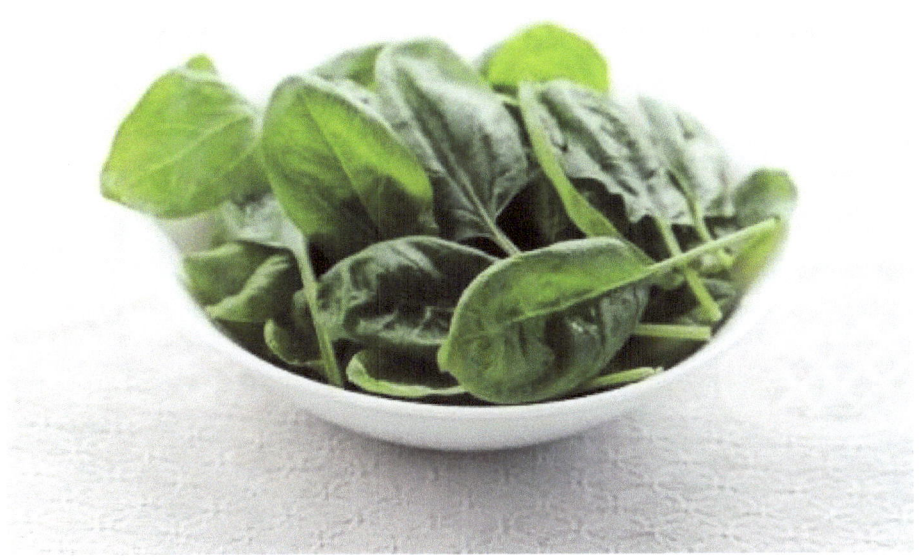

She immediately put me on a diet of fresh liver and freshly cooked spinach in large quantities. Along with that she gave me plenty of red fresh tomatoes, as many as I could eat, deseeded. According to her, every grandmother knew that! Along with that, she also added radish leaves, oranges, apples, beet roots, green leafy vegetables, fenugreek, and pomegranates to my diet. And I soon found myself fit and fine with absolutely no anemia problem ever again.

Remember, if you suffer from any gallstones or any sort of uric acid stone build up in your body, you are not going to eat tomatoes in any form.

Instead, you can try drinking half a cup of fresh beetroot juice, 4 times a day, which is also considered to be a good traditional way of helping patients suffering from leukemia since ancient times.

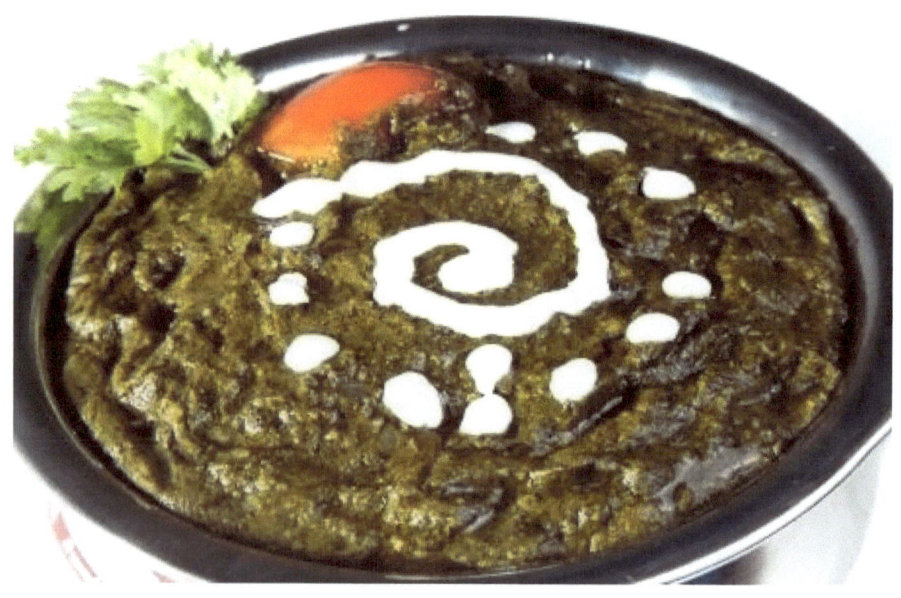

Delicious cooked spinach with tomatoes and cream

Toxic Removing Tonics

In ancient times, people suffering from skin diseases brought about by the accumulation of toxins in the body were given half a glass of fresh carrot juice, before their breakfast and at about 4 o'clock in the evening. 10 days of this treatment and any problem of acne, skin diseases, and toxin buildup in the body would immediately be cured permanently.

Gout

If you are suffering from gout or joint problems, you are going to drink lots of carrot juice, because it equalizes the balance of acids in the body. Gout is normally caused due to a uric acid buildup in the body. This is going to be neutralized and cured with lots of carrots in your diet. Also, if you are suffering from anemia, half a glass of fresh carrot juice is going to increase your RBC count naturally.

In olden times, this juice was given to children in order to prevent them from infections in the eyes, throat, and air passage.

People suffering from flatulence were given carrot juice to get rid of all that accumulated toxin buildup.

Carrots are excellent for keeping your liver toned up, especially if you are suffering from liver and kidney problems, infections in the urinary bladder, prevention of kidney stones, and other such related problems.

In fact, cod liver oil is considered to be an nutritionally equivalent of carrots. Try this experiment. Drink a glass full of carrot juice, before you go to work. And then look at your output before you got tired. You will be surprised to notice that within 2 – 3 months, you were working long hours at a stretch without even feeling the faintest vestiges of tiredness.

Anybody suffering from a vitamin A deficiency would do well to chew upon one carrot every day. Do not peel it.

Carrots for Skin Diseases

I did not know that carrots were good for skin diseases, but I know about a person who had white patches on his neck and chest, and he decided to eat lots of carrots during the fresh carrot season. Within 3 months, all his white patches were gone, and his skin looked healthy and glowing.

I have never heard about this cure for skin diseases, but I have seen this happening. So consider this serendipity, and if you find melanin deficiency occurring anywhere in your body, especially in visible regions, start eating lots of raw carrot. Along with that, drink plenty of carrot juice.

Also, if you are suffering from parasites in the stomach, drink a small glass of carrot juice, with plenty of salt-and-pepper in it at 4 o'clock in the afternoon. This is going to get rid of those parasites.

Carrots for Chest Diseases

Along with that, if you are suffering from a wet cough, drink lots of carrot juice and chew on lots of carrots. This is going to cure you especially when you have lots of accumulated phlegm in your lungs.

In ancient times, carrots were given to those people suffering from congestion of the lungs, cough, and cold.

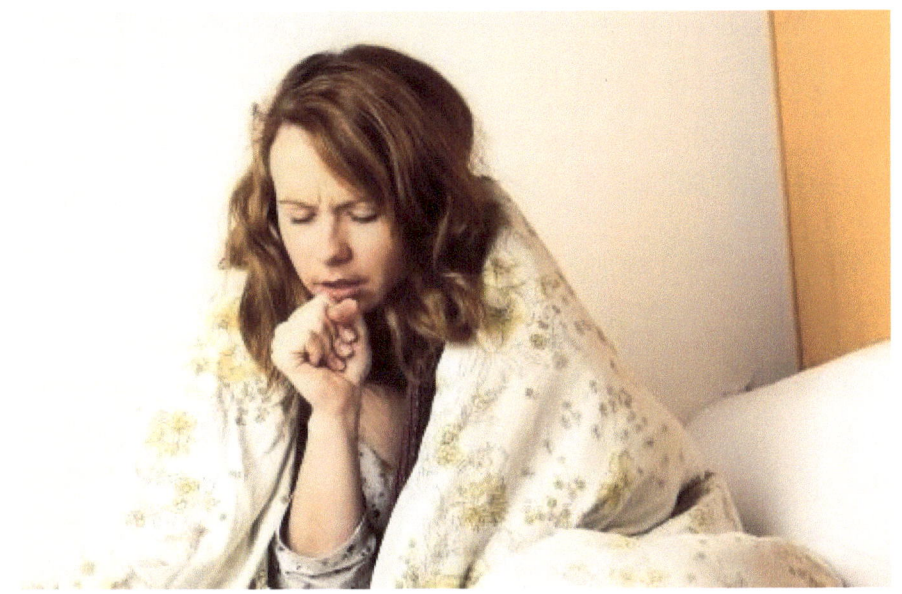

If you are suffering from tonsils and goiter, which is often due to an iodine deficiency, just take a glass of fresh carrot juice every afternoon for 2 – 3 months until you are cured completely. Also, if you add a little bit of cod liver oil, you are going to have quicker results.

Precautions

Remember that when you are taking any diet to add to your blood count, you are going to take these precautions.

You are not going to take any spicy, fried, and rich foods when you are building up your RBC count. In ancient times, cooked food of any sort was not given to the patient. Instead, raw vegetables and raw fruit juice was given in larger quantities to the patient.

In fact, in ancient times the proportion of raw vegetables/fruit to cooked food was eaten in the ratio of 4: 1. This sounds almost unbelievable today because we subsist mainly on cooked food and rarely eat raw vegetables and fruit.

In fact, this proportion was used by the ancients to get rid of chronic diseases in their patients. Do not drink any carrot juice with ice in it.

If you want to add a little bit of spice to your second glass of carrot juice of the day, you would like to add a little bit of ginger, powdered pepper, and rock salt to the juice to make it tastier and more palatable.

You can also eat lots of grated carrots, if you do not want to drink the juice. If you do not want to drink carrot juice in the morning on an empty stomach, you can drink it in the afternoon around 3 – 4 o'clock and just once a day.

How do you get fresh carrot juice?

Traditionally, this was grated on a metal grate. After that, all the pieces were collected in a clean cotton cloth and pressed into a porcelain/glass utensil. The juice was then drunk down immediately. You could also eat the grated carrots for fiber and roughage in your stomach.

Brain Tonics

For this, you need 7 almonds, 7 peppercorns, 2 small cardamoms, 3 g aniseed – this less in the winter and in the summer, you are going to substitute dry coriander seeds instead – soaked in a glass/porcelain utensil overnight.

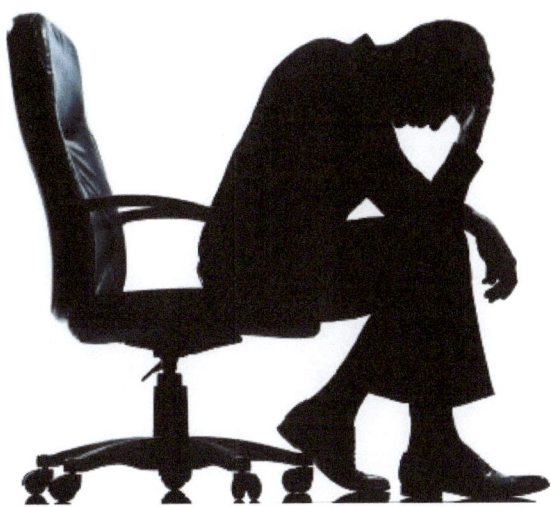

He is stressed and tense. He finds it difficult to concentrate. He needs a natural brain tonic.

Early in the morning, he is going to go out in the fresh air for a walk. Or do some physical exercise. And then he is going to remove the outer covering from the cardamoms, and rub them together into a powder with the peppercorns and the aniseed, until he has a powder.

When he has a thin powder, he is going to filter it. After that he is going to put it in 250 g of water and filter it again. To this he is going to add 2 tablespoons full of honey, and sip it slowly. This is known as almond milk, even though we have not put it in milk. This prevents mental fatigue and helps your concentration.

This was given to all the intellectuals in ancient times, which had to work hard in mental labor, especially students. So if you have a student in the family, give him this tonic and he is never going to suffer from mental fatigue, loss of concentration, absentmindedness, or just any sort of other brain related lethargy.

In the summers, you can try out coriander seeds instead of aniseed, 3 g, 5 – 6 coriander seeds, cold water, and rock candy. In the winter, always use aniseed, warm water, and honey.

You can add or lessen the quantity of the items, depending on the age, size and physique of the person to whom you are feeding this mental tonic, but it is always going to have lots of almonds.

You can then add the number of almonds every week by 2 until the number is anywhere between 13 – 15 almonds. You are going to add to the quantity of the other items proportionately.

In ancient times, children who could not digest their mothers' milk survived on almond milk. So this is the traditional healthy feed from babydom to old age.

When I was young, and was tense because of all the important exams which I had to take, our teachers in our college asked all of us to take fruit, milk, and almond milk for our diet – and nothing else, definitely nothing cooked – and yogurt and honey before we went into the examination room. None of us fell prey to hysterics the moment we saw our question papers. All of us survived exam fever and went on to take higher professional degrees and qualifications.

You could also make a mixture of equal portions of powdered aniseed and rock candy and take 2 tablespoons full with your lunch and with your dinner. Try this for a month or more and see the excellent visible effect on your mental capacities and mental power, 2 months are going to give you the best results.

In ancient times, people suffering from mental weakness and problems were given lots of aniseed to strengthen the brain tissue. Also old people suffering from cataract were given aniseed to prevent the further growth of the cataracts in the eye.

Let me give you a traditional tip, which was used by ancient beauties in order to make their skin fairer in complexion.

They used to take a small fistful – 10 g of aniseeds and chew them thoroughly morning and evening. Not only was this excellent for digestion, but it also made them really fair in complexion.

Grandma's Traditional Gripe Water

Grandma knew how to take care of her little grandchildren from day go itself. That was because all over the world, she used traditional gripe water to prevent colic, stomach problems, cramps, dyspepsia, indigestion, and bringing up milk in their little grandchildren.

She took 6 g of powdered aniseed – 2 teaspoons – and boiled it in a cup of water. When the water had been boiled well, she filtered the water and put it in a glass bottle. One teaspoonful of this gripe water, 2 – 3 times a day and she definitely did not spend lots and lots of money on the modern-day bottled equivalent of gripe water.

So for all those people who think that gripe water is a comparatively modern product to help babies, this water has been around all over the world for millenniums.

Conclusion

This book has given you a large number of traditional healthy tonics and recipes, which have been taken from all over the world and I would not be surprised if your ancestors used them too, wherever you are and in whichever corner you are on the globe.

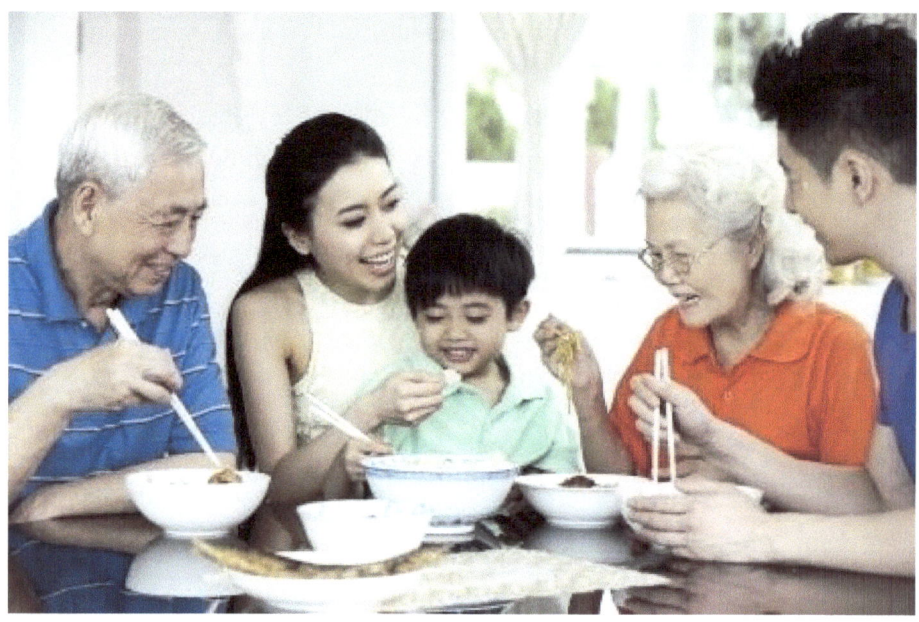

That is because this traditional knowledge was universal and was practiced by the wise women to keep all the members of the family healthy. The mental worker would be fed a mental tonic. Babies and youngsters would be fed health giving tonics. The physical worker would be given tonics which would give him energy and help build tissue and muscles. There were tonics for women and tonics for men. There were tonics for elders too.

So you are going to get one or more natural tonic or food item, which is going to keep you healthy from babyhood to old age.

Stay Healthy, Live Long and Prosper!

Author Bio

Dueep Jyot Singh is a Management and IT Professional who managed to gather Postgraduate qualifications in Management and English and Degrees in Science, French and Education while pursuing different enjoyable career options like being an hospital administrator, IT,SEO and HRD Database Manager/ trainer, movie , radio and TV scriptwriter, theatre artiste and public speaker, lecturer in French, Marketing and Advertising, ex-Editor of Hearts On Fire (now known as Solstice) Books Missouri USA, advice columnist and cartoonist, publisher and Aviation School trainer, ex-moderator on Medico.in, banker, student councilor ,travelogue writer … among other things!

One fine morning, she decided that she had enough of killing herself by Degrees and went back to her first love -- writing. It's more enjoyable! She already has 48 published academic and 14 fiction- in- different- genre books under her belt.

When she is not designing websites or making Graphic design illustrations for clients , she is browsing through old bookshops hunting for treasures, of which she has an enviable collection – including R.L. Stevenson, O.Henry, Dornford Yates, Maurice Walsh, De Maupassant, Victor Hugo, Sapper, C.N. Williamson, "Bartimeus" and the crown of her collection- Dickens "The Old Curiosity Shop," and "Martin Chuzzlewit" and so on… Just call her "Renaissance Woman" - collecting herbal remedies, acting like Universal Helping Hand/Agony Aunt, or escaping to her dear mountains for a bit of exploring, collecting herbs and plants, and trekking.

Check out some of the other JD-Biz Publishing books

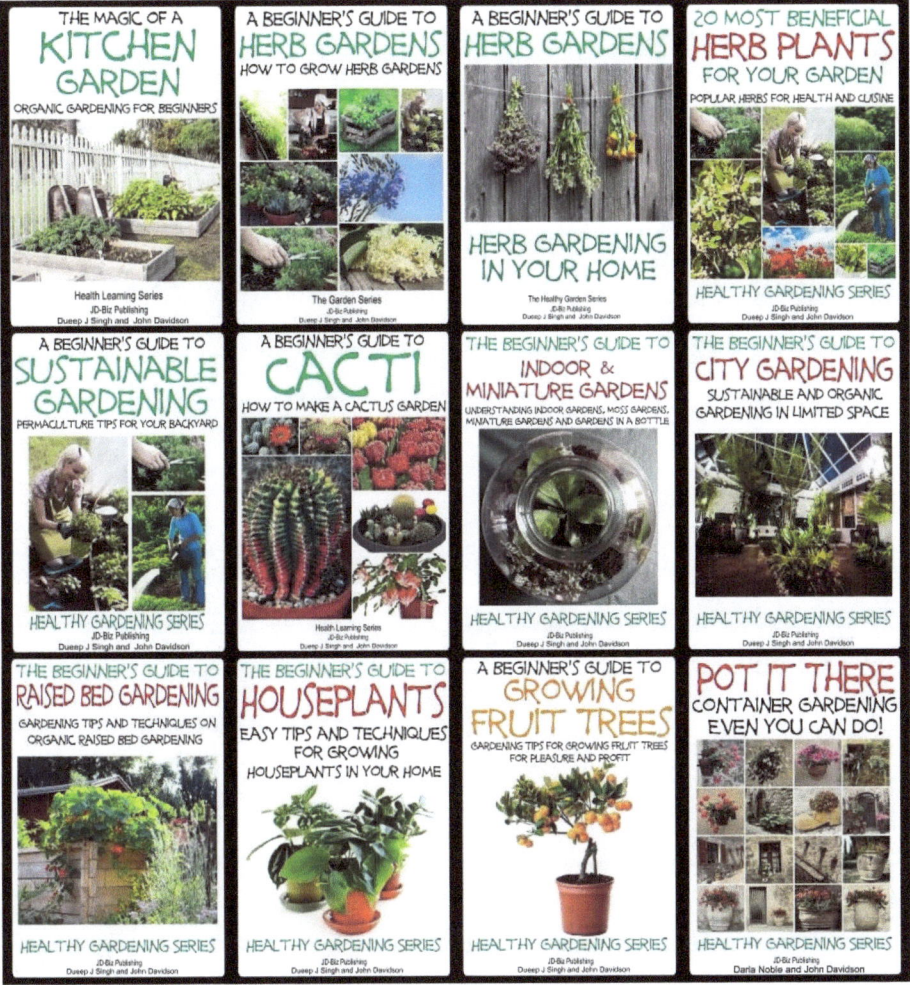

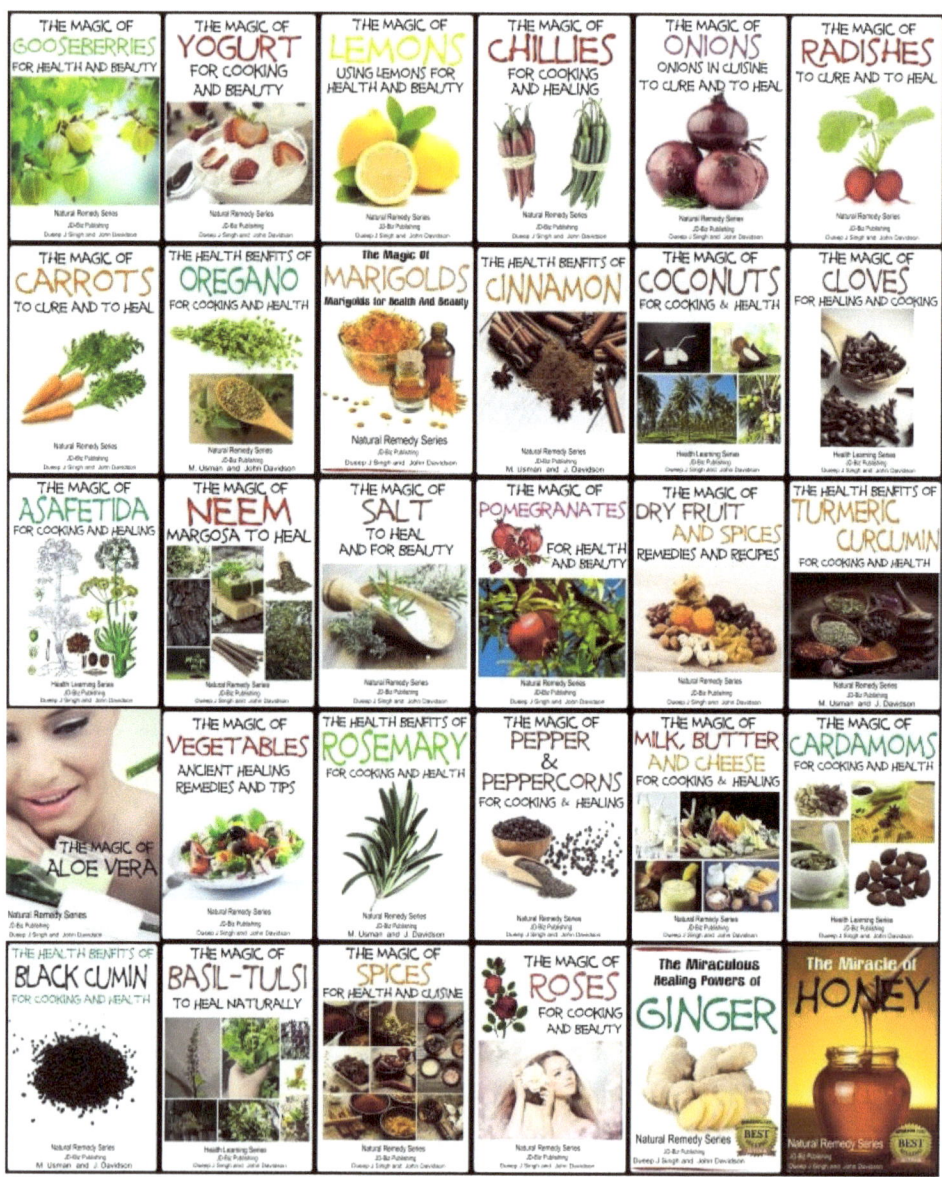

Country Life Books

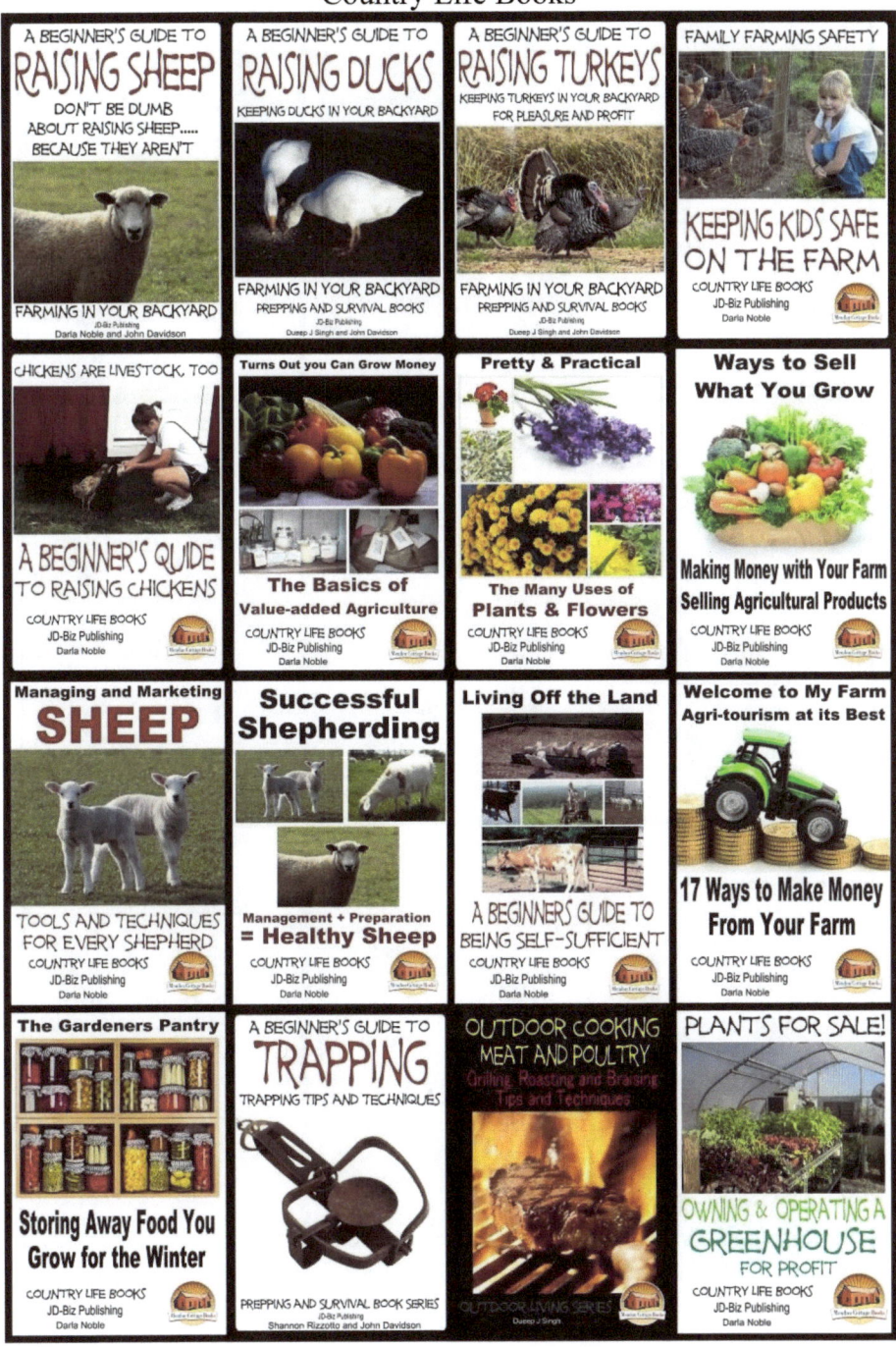

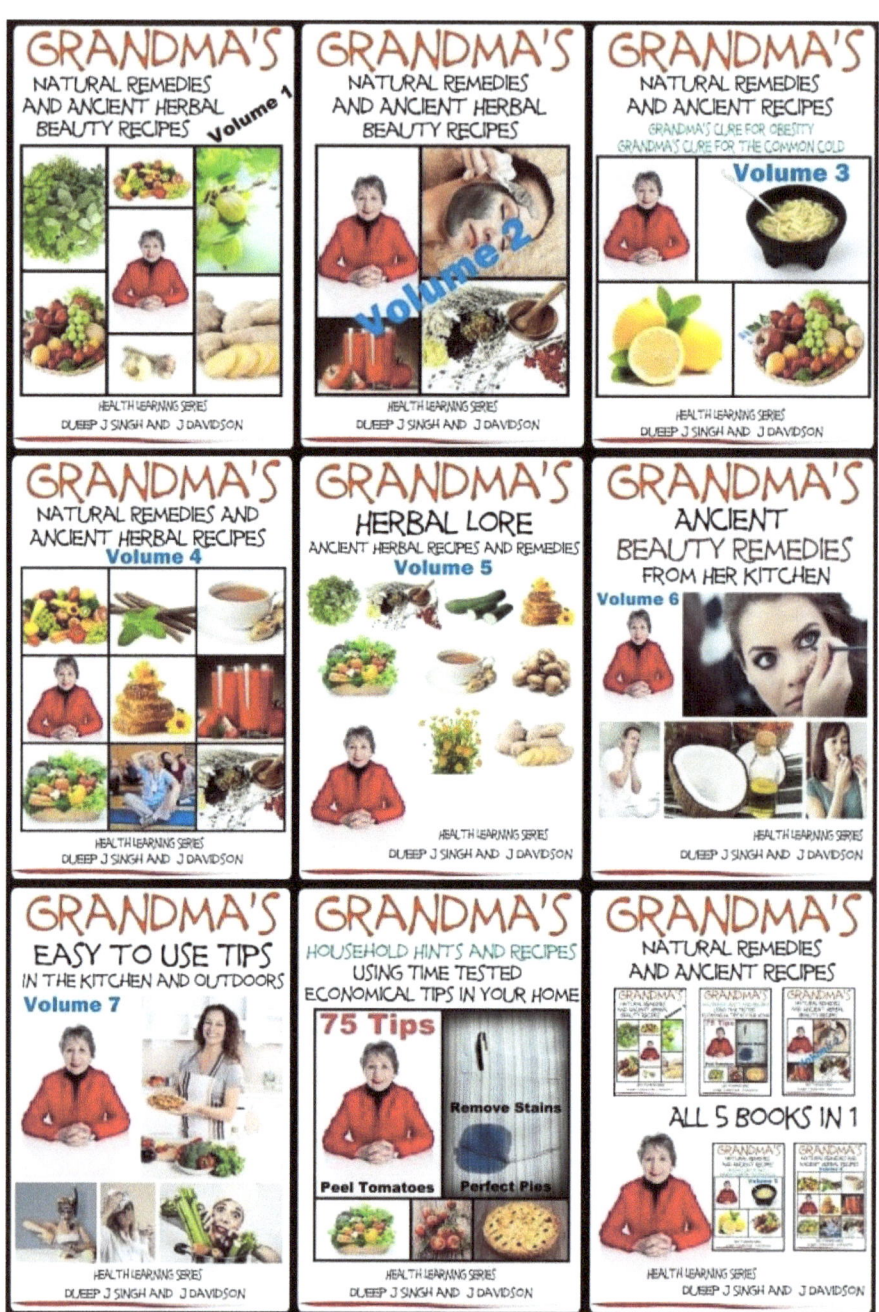

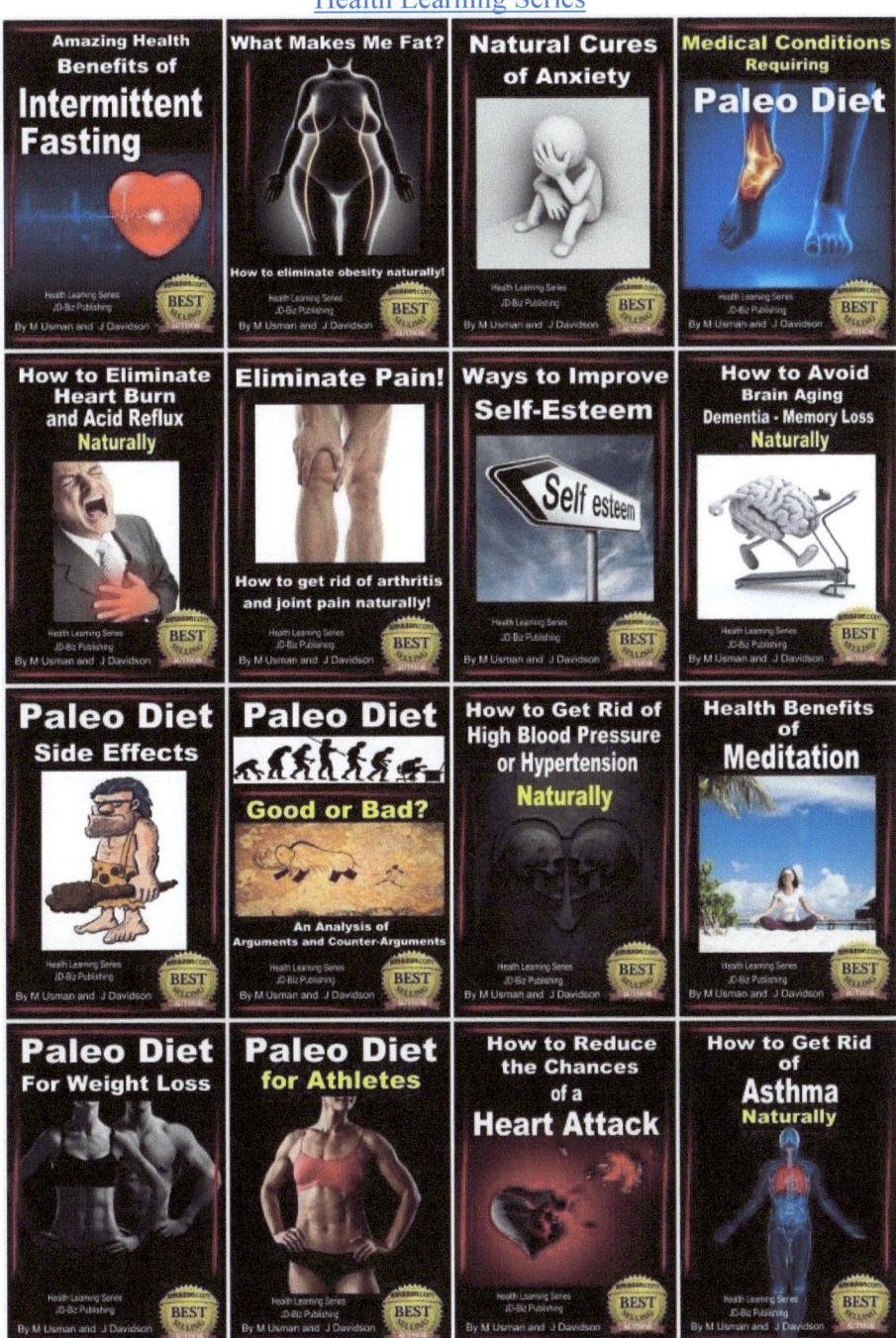

Amazing Animal Book Series

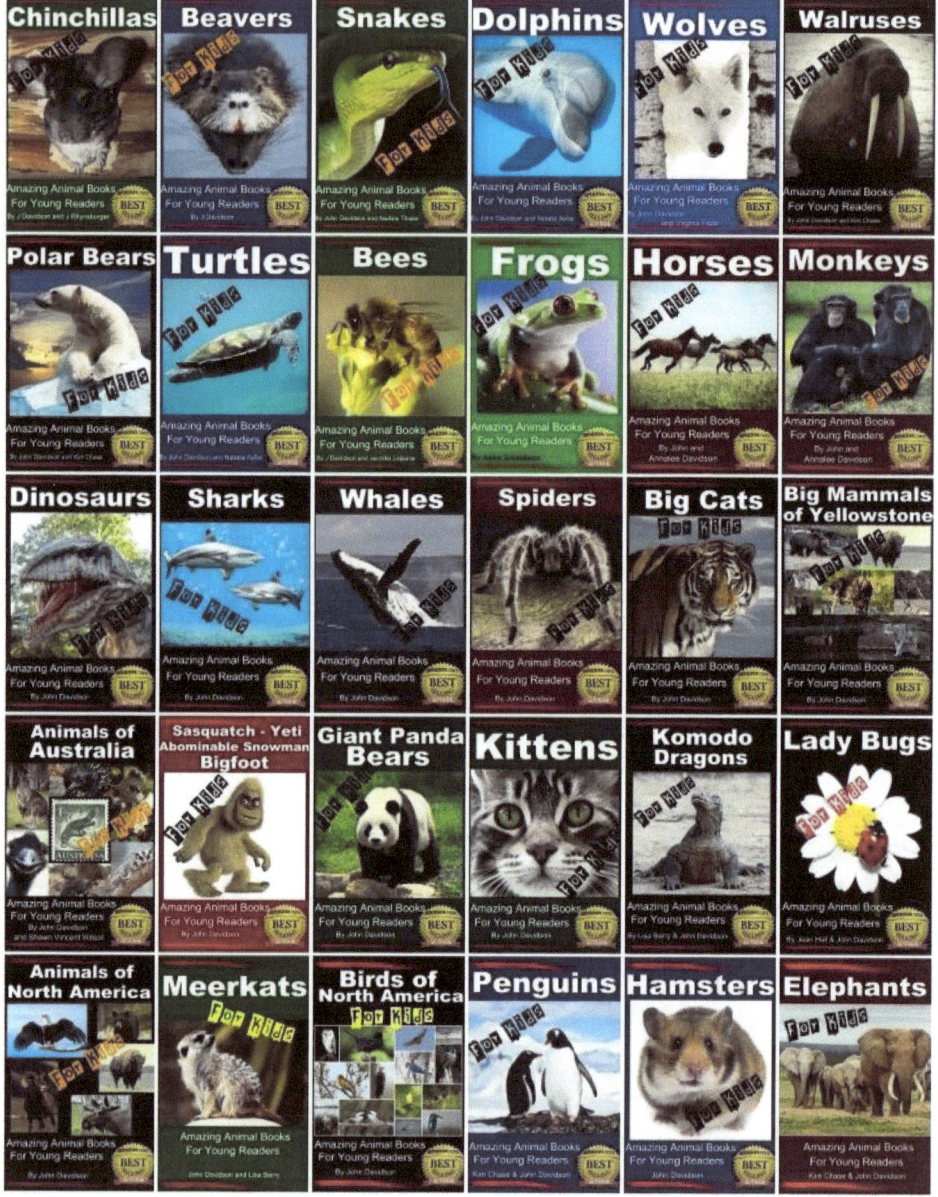

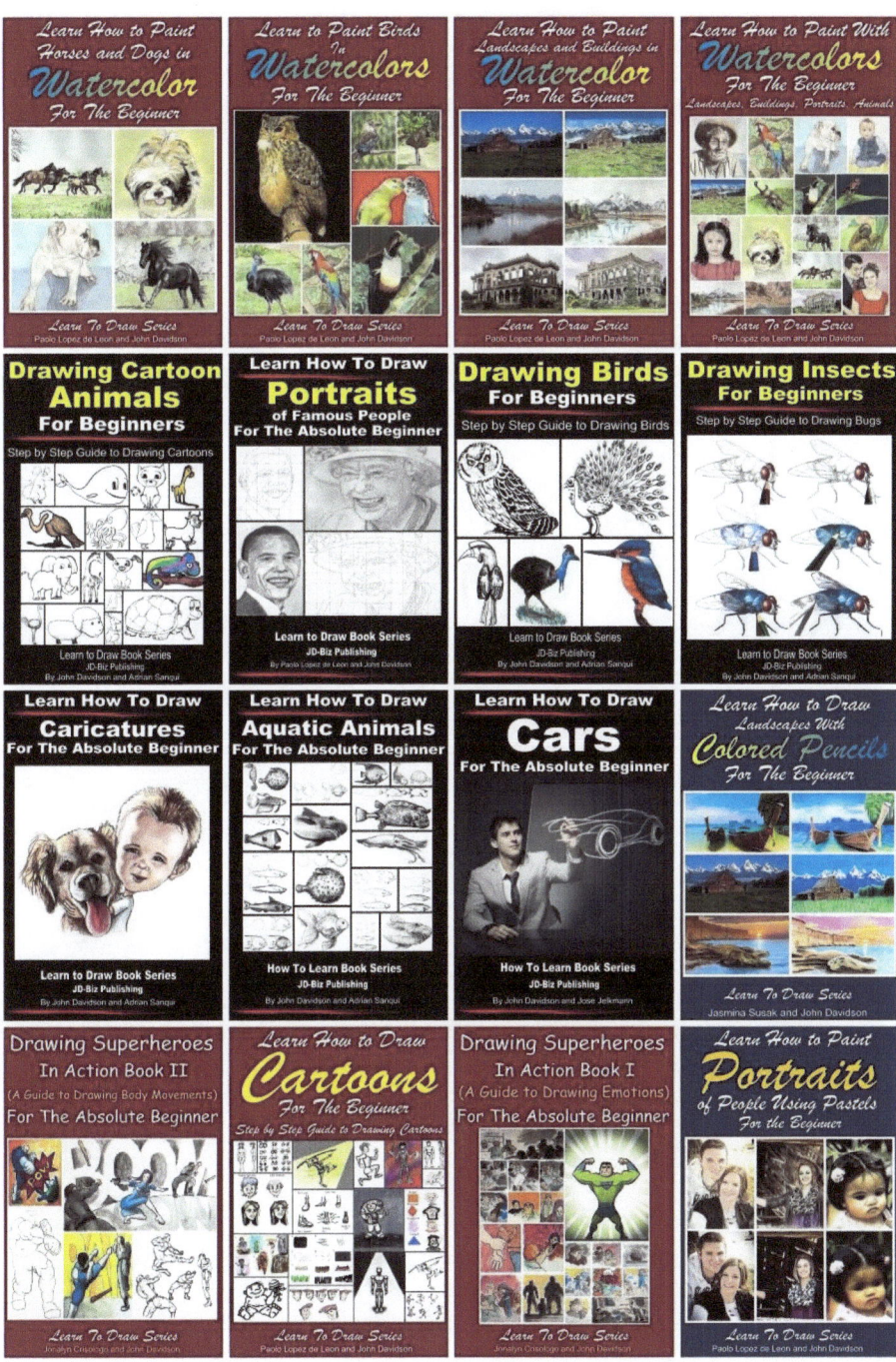

How to Build and Plan Books

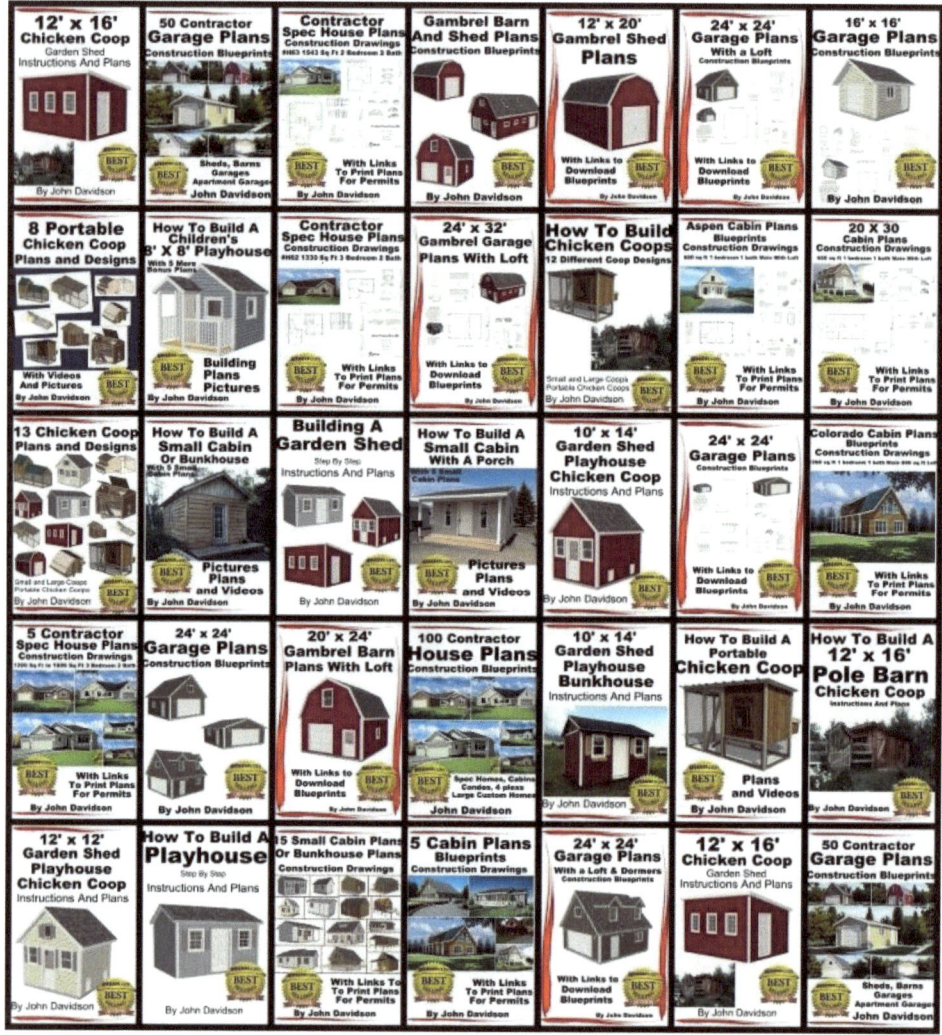

Entrepreneur Book Series

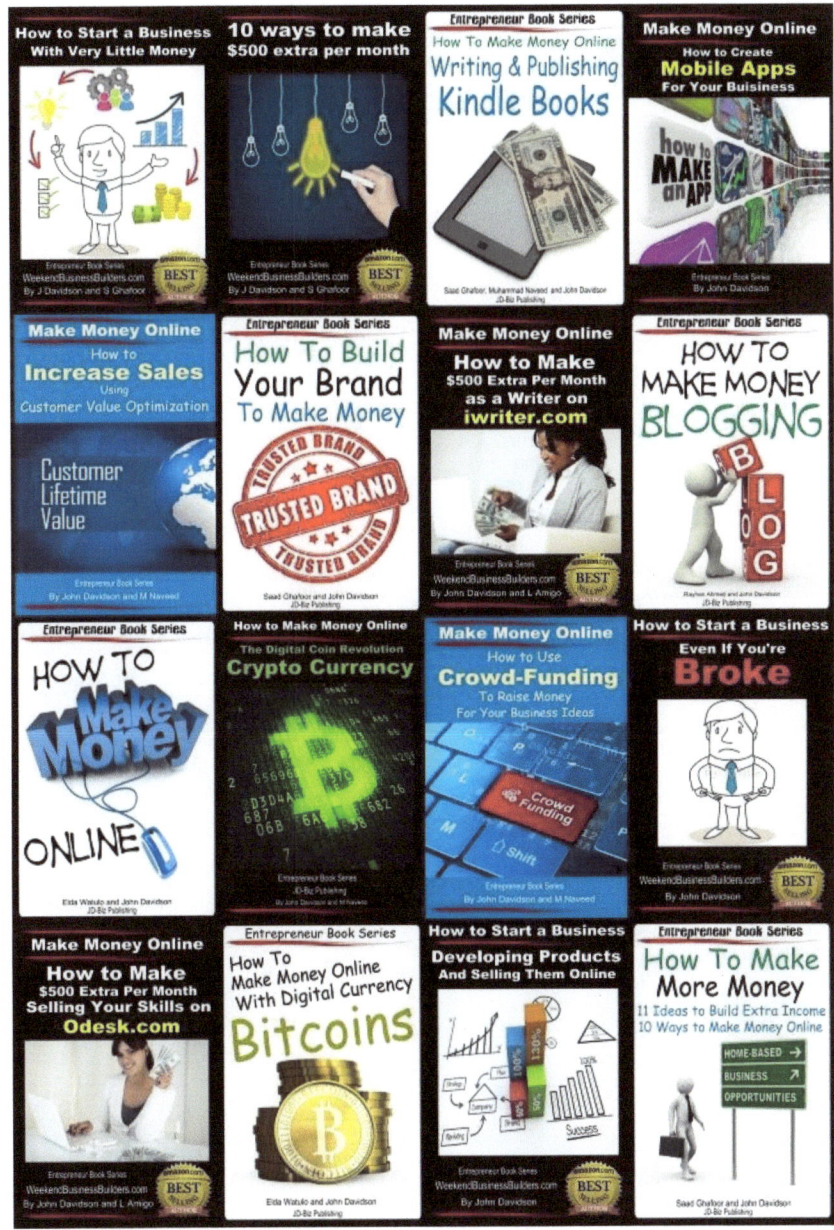

Our books are available at

1. Amazon.com

2. Barnes and Noble

3. Itunes

4. Kobo

5. Smashwords

6. Google Play Books

Download Free Books!

http://MendonCottageBooks.com

Publisher

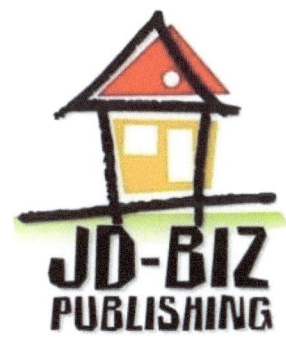

JD-Biz Corp

P O Box 374

Mendon, Utah 84325

http://www.jd-biz.com/

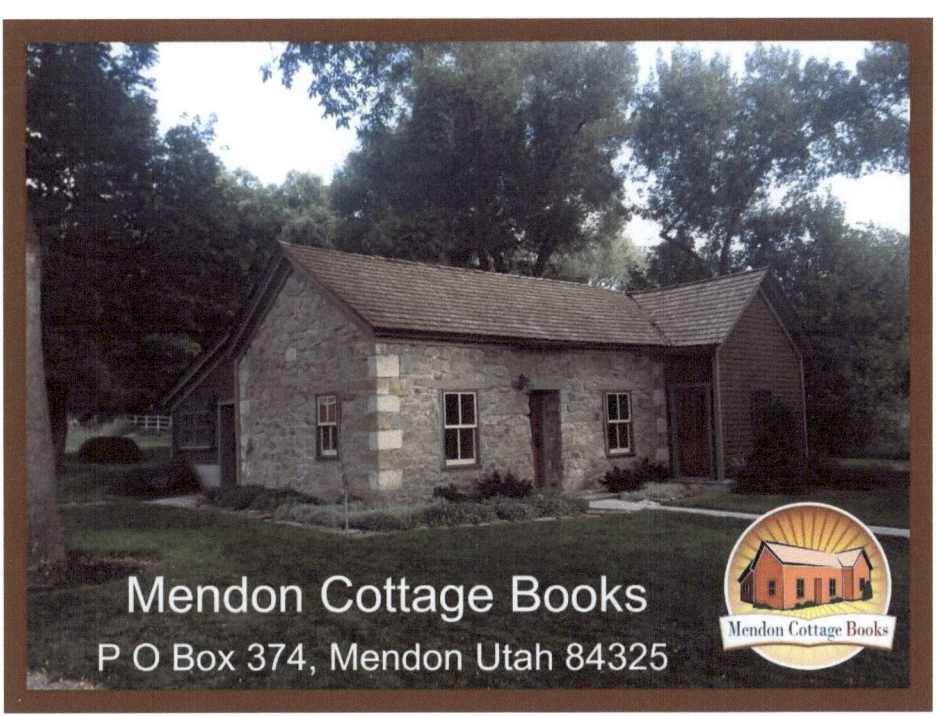

www.ingramcontent.com/pod-product-compliance
Lightning Source LLC
Chambersburg PA
CBHW050832290526
45792CB00001B/357